How To Deal With
Muscle Strain

The Complete Guide To
Strain Management

Dr. Grace Andrews

Table of Contents

Free Gift Inside

Meet the Author, Grace Andrews, DPT.

Doctor of Physical Therapy (DPT) Dr. Grace Andrews is a fervent supporter of musculoskeletal health and rehabilitation. Having worked in the area of physiotherapy for a long time, she offers a wealth of knowledge and skills to help people on their path to muscular health and injury recovery.

Grace's early concern with human mobility and its complex relationship to total well-being led to her devotion to the topic. Her dedication to enhancing recuperation techniques and advocating for prophylactic actions against myofascial tension has garnered her respect from both colleagues and patients.

Her commitment goes beyond providing people with the information and resources needed to properly manage and avoid muscular pain.

Dr. Grace Andrews, the author of this thorough manual on managing muscle strain, hopes to close the knowledge gap between theory and practice by providing readers with a complete method for diagnosing, treating, and avoiding muscular strain for a life enhanced by robust muscle health.

FREE NUTRITIONAL TRACKER INSIDE!!!!

FREE NUTRITIONAL TRACKER INSIDE!!!!

Chapter 1

Understanding Muscle Strain

Muscle strain is a widespread ailment affecting persons of varying ages and physical activity levels. It happens when muscles are exposed to extreme force, resulting in overstretched or damaged muscle fibers.

Whether from rapid movements during sporting activities, carrying large things wrongly, or repeated motions in everyday work, muscular strain presents itself as a prevalent although generally ignored condition.

At its foundation, muscular strain entails structural damage to muscle fibers, causing a variety of symptoms and pain.

The intensity of strain is divided into three grades:

- Mild (Grade I)
- Moderate (Grade II)
- Severe (Grade III)

Each grade delineates the level of muscle fiber injury, determining the severity of symptoms, recovery period, and recommended treatment techniques.

The manifestations of muscular strain involve a variety of symptoms, including regional pain, discomfort, swelling, stiffness, and in extreme instances, bruising or muscle spasms.

Recognizing these symptoms early on assists in rapid action, permitting a more successful treatment plan and a speedier return to regular activities.

Importance of Proper Care

Proper care in controlling muscular strain serves as a vital pillar in the route toward recovery. Timely and suitable therapies not only ease acute symptoms but also play a crucial role in lowering the likelihood of chronic difficulties and long-term repercussions.

The R.I.C.E. protocol—Rest, Ice, Compression, and Elevation—serves as the cornerstone of early therapy, lowering inflammation, relieving discomfort, and supporting the healing process.

Coupled with expert advice from a physiotherapist or healthcare practitioner, individualized treatment regimens and rehabilitation exercises are intended to target the unique type and degree of the strain, accelerating healing and restoring optimum function.

Furthermore, the relevance of preventative efforts cannot be emphasized. Educating folks on adequate warm-up procedures, right body mechanics, and ergonomic modifications in regular tasks dramatically minimizes the risk of muscle strain occurrences.

Integrating these preventive techniques into routines and habits helps as a proactive strategy toward preserving muscle health and avoiding future injuries.

This thorough book acts as a beacon of information, pulling from the experience of physiotherapists, to empower you with detailed insights and concrete techniques.

By improving your awareness of muscle strain and adopting proactive care practices, you empower yourself to successfully manage and overcome this frequent ailment, encouraging prolonged physical well-being and an increased quality of life.

Chapter 2

Anatomy of Muscle Strain

How Muscles Work

Muscles are the workhorses of our body, responsible for movement, stability, and sustaining posture. Understanding their complicated functioning gives significant insights into grasping the mechanics driving muscular tension.

Muscles work by the interaction of contractile units termed sarcomeres, which consist of overlapping actin and myosin filaments. When the body orders a muscle to contract, these filaments glide over one other, shortening the muscle and creating force.

Muscular contraction includes the recruitment of motor units—comprising a motor neuron and the muscle fibers it regulates. Fine motor actions use fewer muscle fibers, whereas bigger motions or lifting heavier weights activate more motor units to provide the needed force output.

The delicate balance of muscular flexibility, strength, and endurance affects their capacity to endure stress and strain. When subjected to excessive force or overloaded above their capability, muscles become prone to strain or damage.

Causes of Muscle Strain

Muscle strain arises from a range of circumstances, frequently happening due to rapid or powerful movements, repeated motions, or insufficient warm-up regimens. Some common reasons include:

1. Overexertion: Engaging in vigorous physical activity without sufficient training or gradually increasing intensity may strain muscles, resulting in tiny rips in the muscle fibers.

2. Poor Body Mechanics: Incorrect posture or inappropriate methods when lifting, bending, or exercising may exert unnecessary stress on muscles, increasing the chance of strain.

3. Lack of Warm-up: Inadequate warm-up procedures or neglecting pre-exercise stretching and preparation fail to prepare muscles for the demands of physical activity, leaving them more sensitive to strain.

4. Fatigue: Prolonged or repeated activity without proper rest periods may tire muscles, decreasing their capacity to absorb shock or withstand tension.

5. Sudden Movements: Swift and sudden movements, particularly when muscles are not conditioned for such motions, may produce strain owing to abrupt stress on the tissues.

6. Previous Injuries: Inadequate therapy or insufficient recovery from earlier muscular injuries will weaken the afflicted region, making it more prone to strain.

Understanding these reasons not only assists in spotting possible risk factors but also stresses the significance of proactive steps in minimizing muscular strain.

By diving into the inner workings of muscles and understanding the varied sources of strain, people may proactively limit the risk of injury, maintaining maximum muscle health and performance.

Chapter 3

Recognizing Muscle Strain

Symptoms and Signs

Identifying the symptoms and indicators of muscular strain is critical for timely intervention and successful therapy.

Common indications include:

1. Localized Pain: A prominent sign of muscular strain, localized pain, generally appears near the location of the injury. The pain may vary from modest discomfort to strong and acute feelings, impacting movement and function.

2. Swelling and Inflammation: In reaction to the damage, the afflicted region may display swelling, redness, and heightened warmth owing to inflammation. This happens when the body commences the healing process, creating fluid collection surrounding the wounded region.

3. Muscle Weakness or Stiffness: Strained muscles may feel weak, making it hard to accomplish everyday motions or tasks. Stiffness and diminished flexibility in the afflicted muscle might also be noticed.

4. Bruising or Discoloration: In more severe cases of muscle strain, bruising or discoloration might occur due to bleeding within the muscle tissues. This usually accompanies a Grade II or III strain.

5. Muscle Spasms: Some individuals might experience involuntary muscle contractions or spasms as a response to the strain, causing additional discomfort.

Differentiating Severity Levels

Understanding the severity of a muscle strain is pivotal in determining the appropriate course of action for treatment and recovery.

The grading system normally comprises three levels:

1. Grade I (Mild): Characterized by minor stretching or microscopic tears within the muscle fibers, Grade I strains usually result in mild pain and minimal loss of function. Recovery is generally quicker, often within a few days to a couple of weeks.

2. Grade II (Moderate): This level involves partial tearing of muscle fibers, leading to more pronounced pain, swelling, and reduced mobility. Recovery may take several weeks, and professional intervention might be necessary to guide rehabilitation.

3. Grade III (Severe): A Grade III strain involves a significant tear or complete rupture of the muscle, causing intense pain, extensive swelling, bruising, and severe impairment in function. Recovery can be prolonged, often requiring extensive rehabilitation and medical attention.

Differentiating these severity levels aids in establishing a specific treatment strategy, selecting the required therapies, and projecting the anticipated recovery schedule for patients afflicted by muscular strain.

Chapter 4

Preventing Muscle Strain

Warm-up and Stretching Techniques

Engaging in correct warm-up exercises and adopting good stretching methods constitute the cornerstone of reducing muscular tension.

These techniques prepare the body for physical exercise, boosting muscular flexibility, circulation, and general performance while lowering the chance of injury.

Warm-up:

A dynamic warm-up technique includes executing low-intensity motions that imitate the activity to come. It progressively increases heart rate, boosts body temperature, and prepares muscles, tendons, and ligaments for more severe effort. Examples include mild running, jumping jacks, or riding.

Stretching:
Static stretching, conducted after a warm-up or physical exercise, includes maintaining a posture that elongates the targeted muscle for a set duration. It promotes flexibility and range of motion, minimizing the chance of muscular tension during exercises. Focus on key muscle groups and hold each stretch for roughly 15-30 seconds without jumping.

Foam Rolling:
Incorporating foam rolling into warm-up exercises helps alleviate muscular tension and enhance blood flow. This self-myofascial release approach targets particular muscle groups, decreasing stiffness and boosting flexibility, hence minimizing the chance of strain.

Dynamic Stretching:
Dynamic stretching comprises controlled motions that take joints and muscles through their complete range of motion. It not only increases flexibility but also primes the muscles for action by simulating the motions of the impending workout or sport.

Correct Body Mechanics

Adopting good body mechanics during everyday activities, workouts, and lifting routines considerably mitigates the risk of muscular strain. Fundamental principles include:

1. Keeping Proper Posture: Whether standing, sitting, or lifting, keeping a neutral spine, proper weight distribution, and avoiding slouching or overextension preserves muscles from unneeded strain.

2. Lifting Techniques: When lifting large things, bend at the knees, maintain the back straight, and lift using the legs rather than the back muscles. Avoid quick jerking actions and distribute weight evenly.

3. Ergonomics: Adjust workstations, seats, and equipment to ergonomically correspond with the body's natural position. This decreases strain during extended sitting or repeated chores.

4. Balanced Exercise Routine: Varying exercise routines and implementing cross-training activities avoid overuse of certain muscle groups, minimizing the risk of discomfort due to repeated stress.

5. Proper Footwear: Wearing suitable footwear matched to the activity or exercise substantially aids in preserving healthy body mechanics. Supportive shoes that offer cushioning and stability lessen stress on the muscles and joints, minimizing the chance of strain.

6. Progressive Training: Progressive rise in intensity and duration during exercise or sporting activities helps muscles, tendons, and ligaments to adapt and strengthen progressively. Avoid rapid jumps in training volume or intensity to avoid overexertion and strain.

7. Rest and Recovery: Adequate rest intervals between exercises or activities help muscles to heal and regenerate. Incorporating regular rest days into workout regimens avoids overuse injuries and enhances muscle repair.

8. Proper Hydration and Nutrition: Staying hydrated and maintaining a balanced diet rich in nutrients, especially those supporting muscular health, assists in muscle rehabilitation and minimizes the risk of fatigue-induced strains.

9. Mindful Movements: Remaining conscious of bodily movements and avoiding rapid, jerky motions or excessive force during exercises considerably minimizes the chance of strain. Focus on smooth, controlled motions to spare muscles from undue tension.

By meticulously incorporating these preventative measures into everyday routines and physical activities, people may successfully decrease the incidence of muscle tension, enhancing overall musculoskeletal health and minimizing the probability of injury.

Chapter 5

Relieving Muscle Tension

The acronym R.I.C.E. stands for "rest, ice, compression, and elevation."

One of the most basic ways to treat muscular tension and speed up the recovery process is using the R.I.C.E. method:

1. Rest:
During the first stage of muscular tension, rest is very necessary. Give the aching muscles a break from activities that make them worse so they can recover. However, full immobility is typically not suggested, since mild movement may help in circulation and avoid stiffness.

2. Ice:
Applying ice to the damaged region helps decrease inflammation, edema, and

discomfort. Use an ice pack or wrap ice in a towel and apply it to the afflicted region for 15-20 minutes every few hours throughout the first 24-48 hours post-injury.

3. Compression:

Compression using an elastic bandage or wrap over the wounded region aids in lowering swelling and gives support to the afflicted muscle. Ensure the compression is snug but not too tight to prevent limiting blood flow.

4. Elevation:

Elevating the damaged location, especially above heart level, assists in lowering edema by permitting appropriate outflow of fluids. This may be performed by propping up the wounded limb on pillows or cushions wherever feasible.

Physical Therapy and Exercises

Once the acute phase of the injury has faded, physical therapy plays a critical role in recovering muscular function, strength, and flexibility.

A skilled physiotherapist may build a personalized rehabilitation program according to the individual's unique ailment and requirements.

Key Components of Physical Therapy:

1. Stretching and Range of Motion Exercises: Gentle stretching exercises assist in enhancing flexibility and restore the muscle's range of motion, reducing stiffness and facilitating recovery.

2. Strengthening Exercises: Gradually adding strengthening exercises targets the injured muscle areas, assisting in regaining strength and endurance. These exercises improve as the injury heals, concentrating on controlled movements to prevent re-injury.

3. Functional Exercises: Functional exercises attempt to emulate everyday activities or sports-specific motions to retrain the afflicted muscles, ensuring they can execute their intended function without strain.

4. Modalities and Techniques: Physiotherapists may apply numerous techniques such as ultrasound, electrical stimulation, or massage to relieve pain, decrease inflammation, and promote tissue recovery.

Adhering to a systematic rehabilitation program under the supervision of a professional assists in a safe and rapid recovery, lowering the risk of repeated strain and encouraging a return to regular activities.

Chapter 6

Recovery and Rehabilitation

Gradual Return to Activities

Returning to normal activities or sports after a muscle strain demands a slow and methodical strategy to ensure complete healing and limit the risk of reinjury:

1. Follow Professional Guidance: Consult with a healthcare physician or physiotherapist to decide the optimum timetable for resuming activities. They will evaluate the amount of healing, facilitate your return, and make advice customized to your unique injury.

2. Progressive Resumption: Begin with low-impact or non-strenuous exercises that do not increase discomfort. Gradually increase the intensity, length, and complexity of exercises as the damaged muscle develops strength and flexibility.

3. Pay Attention to Warning Signs: During the slow return, keep attentive for any indicators of discomfort, pain, or weakness. If sensations persist or worsen, it can suggest that the muscle has not recovered, indicating the need to cut down activity levels.

4. Focus on Technique and Form: Emphasize good body mechanics, posture, and technique when participating in activities to avoid tension on the recovering muscle. Avoid overexertion and heed to your body's warnings to avoid setbacks in recovery.

Preventing Recurrence

Preventing the recurrence of muscular strain entails adopting preventive measures and lifestyle modifications to limit future risks:

1. Maintain Conditioning and Strength: Continue with a suitable workout plan that focuses on general strength, flexibility, and conditioning of the muscles. This helps reinforce the muscles, minimizing susceptibility to tension.

2. Regular Warm-ups and Stretching: Prioritize pre-activity warm-up routines and stretching exercises to prepare muscles for effort and limit the chance of strain during physical activities.

3. Proper Nutrition and Hydration: Ensure proper hydration and maintain a balanced diet rich in nutrients important for muscular function and recovery. A proper diet stimulates muscle regeneration and lowers tiredness, minimizing the probability of strain.

4. Listen to Your Body: Be vigilant to any warning signals of impending strain, such as muscular tightness, soreness, or exhaustion. Address these signs quickly by adjusting activity or obtaining expert help to avoid future damage.

5. Periodic Rest and Recovery: Incorporate enough rest times between exercises to provide muscles time to heal and mend. Avoid overtraining or pushing through extreme weariness, since it increases sensitivity to strain.

By applying these techniques, people may considerably lower the risk of recurring muscular strain, promoting a sustainable and injury-free involvement in physical activities and everyday routines.

Chapter 7

Nutrition and Muscle Health

Diet's Role in Muscle Recovery

A balanced and nutrient-rich diet plays a crucial role in muscle rehabilitation, delivering necessary nutrients to promote tissue repair, development, and general muscle health:

1. Protein for Muscle Repair: Proteins, made of amino acids, are necessary for mending damaged muscle tissues following exertion. Consuming enough protein sources such as lean meats, fish, poultry, dairy, legumes, and plant-based sources like tofu or quinoa benefits muscle healing and adaptation.

2. Carbohydrates for Energy Replenishment: Carbohydrates serve as the major energy source during physical activity and aid in rebuilding glycogen reserves in muscles post-exercise. Whole grains, fruits, vegetables, and legumes give prolonged energy and assist in the recuperation process.

3. Healthy Fats for Inflammation Reduction: Incorporating good fats like omega-3 fatty acids found in fatty fish, nuts, seeds, and olive oil will help decrease inflammation, helping the healing process after muscular tension.

4. Hydration for Tissue Repair: Adequate hydration is required for proper nutrition delivery and waste elimination from cells. Proper hydration provides an ideal environment for tissue healing and improves general muscular performance.

Supplements and Their Impact

Supplements may complement a well-rounded diet, giving extra support for muscle repair and health. However, their influence varies, and their use should be directed by individual requirements and expert advice:

1. Protein Supplements: Whey protein, casein, or plant-based protein powders might be practical solutions to augment protein consumption, especially for persons wanting more protein for muscle repair or those with dietary constraints.

2. Branched-Chain Amino Acids (BCAAs): BCAAs, composed of essential amino acids (leucine, isoleucine, and valine), are considered to assist muscle repair and minimize muscular pain post-exercise. They are available in supplement form but may also be taken from food sources including meat, dairy, and legumes.

3. Creatine: Creatine supplements may boost muscular strength and workout performance, assisting in recuperation and adaptation. They are often utilized among athletes and those involved in high-intensity activities.

4. Omega-3 Fatty Acids: Supplementing with omega-3 fatty acids may boost anti-inflammatory mechanisms in the body, possibly lowering inflammation linked with muscular strain and assisting in recovery.

While supplements may be useful, it's vital to emphasize a balanced diet as the major source of nutrients and check with a healthcare practitioner or a certified dietitian before adopting supplements, ensuring they correspond with individual health requirements and objectives.

Chapter 8

Lifestyle Adjustments

Ergonomics in Daily Activities

Ergonomics includes structuring the environment to suit the person, improving comfort, and efficiency, and lowering the danger of strain or injury during everyday activities:

1. Workspace Ergonomics: Ensure correct alignment of workstations by modifying chair height, and desk arrangement, and monitor position to preserve neutral postures. This lowers tension on muscles, notably in the back, neck, and shoulders, lowering the chance of overuse problems.

2. Proper Lifting Techniques: Adopt ideal lifting postures by bending the knees, keeping the back straight, and utilizing the leg muscles to lift large things. Distribute weight evenly and prevent quick, jerky motions that might strain muscles.

3. Supportive Equipment: Utilize ergonomic gear and equipment such as supporting seats, ergonomic keyboards, and mousepads to alleviate strain on muscles and joints during prolonged durations of usage.

4. Breaks and Movement: Incorporate frequent pauses and movements into sedentary work. Stand up, stretch, and change positions periodically to minimize muscular stiffness and lower the risk of strain associated with extended sitting.

Stress Reduction Techniques

Chronic stress may worsen muscular tension and raise the risk of strain. Employing stress reduction strategies may reduce muscular tension and improve relaxation:

1. Mindfulness and Meditation: Practice mindfulness practices, such as meditation or deep breathing exercises, to lower stress levels, relax muscles, and promote general well-being. These activities may reduce muscular tension and enhance resistance to shocks.

2. Regular Exercise and Physical Activity: Engage in regular physical activity or exercises like yoga, tai chi, or aerobic activities to release endorphins and alleviate muscular tension linked with stress. Exercise also helps boost mood and improves relaxation.

3. Time Management and Prioritization: Manage time wisely by prioritizing chores and creating realistic objectives. Avoid overcommitment and practice saying 'no' when required to minimize excessive stress levels that may lead to muscular strain.

4. Healthy Lifestyle Choices: Adopting a healthy lifestyle, including balanced eating, appropriate sleep, and reducing substance usage like coffee or alcohol, favorably influences stress levels, encouraging muscular relaxation and general well-being.

5. Seeking Support: Talking to friends, family, or a professional counselor may give emotional support and coping methods to handle stress efficiently, lessening its influence on muscular tension and strain.

Incorporating these lifestyle improvements into everyday activities fosters a more ergonomic and stress-resilient environment, minimizing the risk of muscular strain and boosting overall physical and mental well-being.

Chapter 9

Special Considerations

Muscle Strain in Different Age Groups

1. Children and Adolescents:

- Growing children and teenagers could be prone to muscular tension due to fast development and engagement in sports activities. Emphasize correct warm-ups, steady development in exercise, and enough rest to reduce tension in growing muscles and growth plates.

2. Adults:

- Adults engaged in physically demanding employment or high-intensity workouts are subject to muscular strain. Proper warm-ups, frequent stretching, and attention to ergonomic principles can decrease the risk of strain, particularly in the back, shoulders, and neck.

3. Seniors:

- Aging muscles tend to lose flexibility and strength, leaving them more sensitive to strain. Encourage mild workouts, such as swimming or tai chi, to maintain muscular flexibility and strength while limiting the chance of strain or injury.

Dealing with Chronic Muscle Strain

Chronic muscular strain refers to repeated or chronic tension in certain muscle groups, frequently needing specialist care and management:

1. Professional Assessment:

- Seek examination by a healthcare expert, physiotherapist, or sports medicine specialist to discover underlying reasons, diagnose muscular imbalances, and devise an appropriate treatment strategy.

2. Targeted Rehabilitation:

- Engage in a tailored rehabilitation program concentrating on strengthening weak muscles, increasing flexibility, and resolving imbalances to reduce chronic strain and avoid future episodes.

3. Activity Modification:

- Modify activities or workouts that routinely induce muscular tension. Adjust intensity, duration, or technique to decrease tension on afflicted muscles and enhance recuperation.

4. Consistent Self-Care:

- Adhere to continuous self-care measures, including good warm-ups, enough rest, stretching, and utilizing supporting equipment or braces if suggested, to manage chronic strain and avoid aggravation.

5. Address Underlying Factors:

- Address any contributory factors such as bad posture, repeated motions, or overtraining. Modify living patterns and use ergonomic concepts to lessen pressure on muscles.

Managing chronic muscular strain demands a diverse strategy, including focused rehabilitation, activity adjustment, and proactive self-care measures suited to the individual's requirements and circumstances.

Chapter 10

Conclusion

In the search for understanding and controlling muscular tension, this comprehensive book acts as a light of information, giving insights, techniques, and professional guidance from the domain of physiotherapy and musculoskeletal health.

Throughout these pages, we've studied the many facets of muscle strain, equipping you with the skills and knowledge required to handle this widespread ailment.

From knowing the architecture of muscular strain to detecting its symptoms, classifying severity levels, and using the R.I.C.E. approach for early therapy, every element of treating muscle strain has been painstakingly explored.

The relevance of adequate treatment, including physical therapy, personalized exercises, and a gradual return to activities, has been stressed to assist in optimum recovery.

Moreover, this book goes beyond therapy to incorporate preventative measures, addressing ergonomics, stress reduction strategies, and the critical function of nutrition in muscle health.

By looking into unique concerns for distinct age groups and chronic muscular strain, we've underlined the importance of specialized therapies to meet varied life phases and persistent difficulties.

The road toward efficiently coping with muscle tension does not finish here; it continues to be a proactive and comprehensive approach to total muscle well-being. It is a path focused on awareness, prevention, and developing a lifestyle favorable to sustaining maximum muscle health.

As you begin on this path, remember that each step taken—whether in warm-up routines, mindful movements, or seeking expert guidance—contributes to the robust health of your muscles.

By accepting the ideas put forth in this book and integrating them into your everyday life, you pave the road for prolonged muscular health and an empowered, injury-resistant existence.

May this book serve as a complete resource and a companion in your search for robust muscles, encouraging a life enhanced by physical well-being and an ongoing pursuit of active, pain-free living.

Nutrition is the cornerstone of muscle recovery—a vital fuel that rebuilds, replenishes, and shapes the path to strength and endurance.""Nutrition is the cornerstone of muscle recovery—a vital fuel that rebuilds, replenishes, and shapes the path to strength and endurance.

My Daily
Nutrition

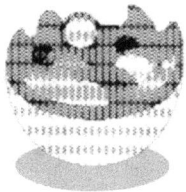

Name: _____   Date: _____

Breakfast

Lunch

Dinner

Grocery List

- _____
- _____
- _____
- _____
- _____
- _____
- _____

Nutrition

Notes

My Daily Nutrition

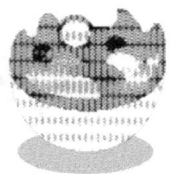

Name: _____ Date: _____

Breakfast	Lunch	Dinner

Grocery List

- _____
- _____
- _____
- _____
- _____
- _____
- _____

Nutrition

Notes

My Daily
Nutrition

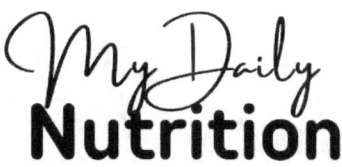 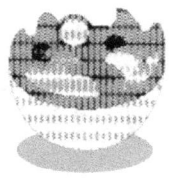

Name: _____ Date: _____

Breakfast	Lunch	Dinner

Grocery List

- _____
- _____
- _____
- _____
- _____
- _____
- _____

Nutrition

Notes

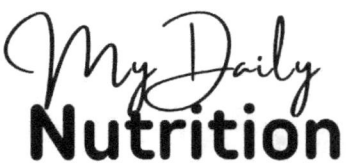 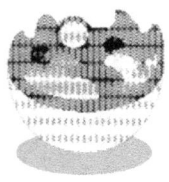

My Daily
Nutrition

Name: _____ Date: _____

Breakfast	Lunch	Dinner

Grocery List

- _____
- _____
- _____
- _____
- _____
- _____
- _____

Nutrition

Notes

My Daily
Nutrition

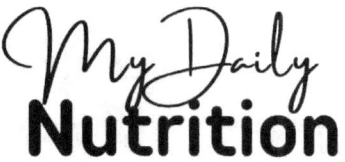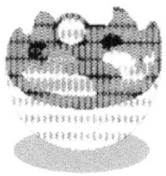

Name: _____   Date: _____

Breakfast	Lunch	Dinner

Grocery List

- _____
- _____
- _____
- _____
- _____
- _____
- _____

Nutrition

Notes

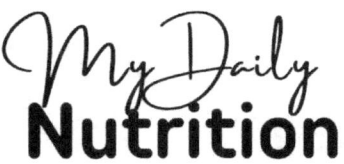 **My Daily** **Nutrition**

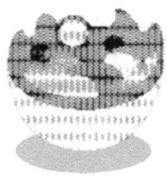

Name: _____ Date: _____

Breakfast

Lunch

Dinner

Grocery List

- _____
- _____
- _____
- _____
- _____
- _____
- _____

Nutrition

Notes

My Daily
Nutrition

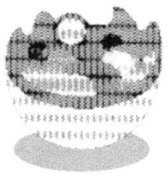

Name: _____ Date: _____

Breakfast	Lunch	Dinner

Grocery List

- _____
- _____
- _____
- _____
- _____
- _____
- _____

Nutrition

Notes

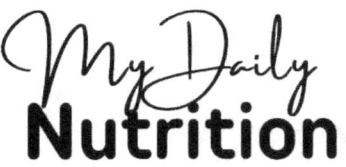 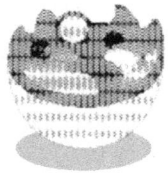

My Daily
Nutrition

Name: _____   Date: _____

Breakfast	Lunch	Dinner

Grocery List

- _____
- _____
- _____
- _____
- _____
- _____
- _____

Nutrition

Notes

My Daily
Nutrition

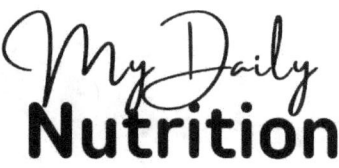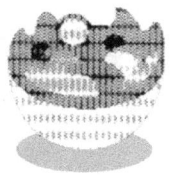

Name: _____   Date: _____

Breakfast	Lunch	Dinner

Grocery List

- _____
- _____
- _____
- _____
- _____
- _____
- _____

Nutrition

Notes

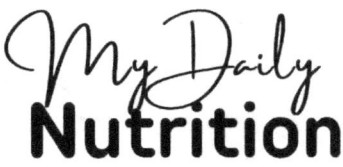 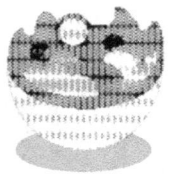

My Daily Nutrition

Name: _____ Date: _____

Breakfast	Lunch	Dinner

Grocery List

- _____
- _____
- _____
- _____
- _____
- _____
- _____

Nutrition

Notes

www.ingramcontent.com/pod-product-compliance
Lightning Source LLC
Chambersburg PA
CBHW062253290526
45794CB00006B/2526